MW01697939

Living with Depressive Illness and Finding Joy Again

Living with Depressive Illness and Finding Joy Again

A Holistic Approach

Edward "Ted" Dunn

VANTAGE PRESS
New York

The opinions and instructions expressed herein are solely those of the author. Each individual should seek the advice of his or her medical professional before starting any new medical program.

Cover design by Susan Thomas

FIRST EDITION

Published by Vantage Press, Inc.
419 Park Ave. South, New York, NY 10016

Manufactured in the United States of America
ISBN: 0-533-15113-9

Library of Congress Catalog Card No.: 2004099547

0 9 8 7 6 5 4 3 2 1

I dedicate this book to the following persons: to my father who taught me to love life and trust the world even though he only lived for 7 1/2 years into my life. Secondly, I dedicate it to my hero, my mother, who cared for us children through the death of my father in 1927, through the death of my brother at age six, in 1928, and through the Great Depression after 1929. Somehow she found the vision and courage to see my remaining sister (Syracuse University—Phi Beta Kappa) and brother (Colgate and Yale Law) through college and prepared for life, while living as a widow for fifty-six years. My other primary hero and loved one was my wife, Ann, who was my best friend for sixty-three years and my wife for sixty years. She supported me through many years that included both the times when I experienced rapture and discontent. Then, there is our daughter, son-in-law, and grandson, who have all been inspirational for me. Finally, I thank the relatives, teachers, coaches, students, and friends who have shared in my journey.

Contents

Living with Depressive Illness and Finding Joy Again

I

My Credibility (E.T. Dunn) as This Author

I am not a psychiatrist and I have no degree in psychology. However, I do have some credentials that encourage me to write on this topic, as follows:

I have experienced a significant amount of depression in my life. This started with a possible family genetic disposition to this illness and as an early-life experience, where I was involved with the death of my father. The genetic factor involves my knowledge of the suicide of a first cousin, at a relatively early age, following a setback in his life. The involvement in my father's (and brother's) deaths are described in my book, *What Is This Thing Called Love,* (1996) in the following words:

> My father owned four farms in central New York devoted to a pea and bean business. One day in June 1927, when I went with him to taxi local pickers, was destined for tragedy. I was seven and one half years old at the time, and I have blocked much of the details of the event from my mind. My father stopped at a home near the railroad station to get a local picker. I waited in the passenger side of the front seat of the Studebaker, while he went to the door of the home. When he returned and the person had gotten in the backseat, my father attempted to start the car.
>
> The car would not start. This was often the case in

those days, so he got out to crank the car. Tragically, it had not been put into neutral but had been left in gear. In those days the big shift gear handle came out of the floorboard. Further, the big-handled emergency brake was not set, to my knowledge. As a result, when he cranked the car from the front, it jumped forward when it started, knocked him down, and rolled onto his body. He died later that day of internal injuries.

My memory is incomplete, but I read years later, in a newspaper account my mother had saved, that I moved over and got my foot on the foot brake as soon as I realized the car was moving forward. It was too late to save my father's life. For years, I wondered if I might have played with the gear shift while my father was away from the car. Recently, a friend reminded me I would have needed to press the clutch down to change the gears.

The impact of my involvement in my father's death has had a lifetime effect on my attitude and actions. Looking back, I believe I have had a low level of depression for most of my life due to a feeling of loneliness for my loving father. Further, I have had somewhat of a lover's quarrel with the world. My father and mother taught me by their actions to love and trust the world during my formative years of life. However, this love and trust was wounded by my father's death experience. As the years passed by, I took solace from the fact that he did not want to leave us. Mother's great love and sense of humor helped immensely as well. She was also a classical pianist and had a trained voice. Her near daily music sessions, also helped us balance our grief. Following Father's death, we four children were taken by relatives and we did not attend the wake or the funeral. This was done to protect us. I've come to appreciate this action, as that was more a custom with young children following a death in the family in those days. Today, children are encouraged to share more in the grieving process, which I believe is better. I do remember crying hysterically immediately after my father's accident, when I was taken into a nearby home and attempts were made by kind neighbors to comfort me. Beyond that I would not bring the subject up to anyone for many years, even into the early years of my marriage.

My father's sudden tragic death was not the end of our family tragedy. My mother was left with four children: Dorothy (Dot, age nine), Edward Jr. (Ted, age seven), Peter (age five), and William (Win, age two). Years later Mother told me that she vowed at my father's death to "never be afraid again." Mother's courage was severely tested again in 1928 when Peter died within a week after developing what was called the croup, an often lethal bronchial infection. Today it could most likely be readily cured, but this was not the case with dear little Peter.

My first major depression came at age fifty following a deep involvement in the Civil Rights period at Springfield College, Springfield, MA. I was a full professor of health and physical education and head football coach. It was a time that saw the Springfield College family deeply disturbed and divided over the issue of Black students' civil rights. I had been in the segregated Army Air Corps for thirty-nine months in World War II and felt a strong need to be involved in trying to settle these divisive issues peacefully and fairly. As a result I volunteered and was elected co-chairperson of the Springfield College Collegian, called for by the President, during the summer of 1970. This was a thirty-five person group of alumni, board of trustees, faculty, administrators, staff, and student representatives, which met nearly every day on campus during the summer of 1970. (The students said you could tell the trustees because they wore ties.)

This was a wrenching experience for all involved. It did lead to a new college governance system based on improved democratic principles and reasonably fair "middle of the road" decisions regarding present and future civil rights policies at this College. There were extremists at either end of the controversy over how to react to the demands of the Black students. Some wanted to meet their every demand. Some didn't want to meet any of them and to just dismiss them from the college as they were disruptive. Some Springfield College family members considered the Collegian members (including myself) disloyal to the college tradition if they differed in their position. I went from this experience directly into teaching and coaching football in the fall of 1970. This was emotion on top of emotion.

This depressive episode following the 1970 football season, caused me to go on medication and involvement in talk therapy with a psychiatrist. I found joy again in six months due to these treatments, the great love of my wife, Ann, family friends and my own efforts, described in a following chapter.

Further experiences that help me to feel I can write on this topic are:

The three added similar experiences, to this initial clinical depression. These took place when I made the difficult decision to retire seven years before it was required (1983) as a full tenured professor. This was followed by another episode after diagnosis with prostrate cancer (1989) and by the death of my wife after nearly sixty years of marriage (2001). Each of the first two of these depressive times lasted six months while the one following Ann's death lasted eighteen months before I went off medication and professional psychotherapy. I also studied mental health and illness when completing doctoral program in health education at Boston University and the teaching in this area at Springfield College.

Further, I have volunteered for eighteen years with the

National Alliance for the Mentally Ill of Western Massachusetts, and am presently an honorary life member. I also volunteered for ten years with the Springfield Citizens Advocacy Project, which is devoted to creating a one-on-one relationship between a volunteer and a person with a mental illness. In these experiences I have read extensively on the subject of mental illness, attended dozens of educational meetings on this topic and observed first hand many persons who are coping with this disease. Finally, I served as a friend for ten years with a former college student who was in my class. He became challenged with a severe mental illness after his freshman year of college when he had no family assistance, as his mother was deceased and his father was an abusive alcoholic.

II

The Nature and Scope of Depression

What Is a Depressive Disorder?

A depressed disorder is an illness that involves the body, mood and thoughts. It affects the way a person eats and sleeps, the way one feels about oneself and the way one thinks about things. A depressive disorder is not the same a passing blue mood, or the sign of a personal weakness, or a condition that can be wished away . . . without treatment symptoms can last for weeks, months or years. *Appropriate treatment today can help most people who suffer from depression.*

—(National Institute of
Mental Health [NIH],
Publication No. 004501
Year 2000)

In any given one-year period, 9.5 percent of the population, or about 18.8 million American adults, suffer from a depressive illness. The economic cost for this disorder is high, but the cost in human suffering cannot be estimated. Depressive illnesses often interfere with normal functioning and cause pain and suffering not only to those who have a disorder, but also to those who care about them. Serious depression can destroy family life, as well as the life of the ill person. But much of this suffering is unnecessary.

Most people with depressive illness do not seek treatment, although the great majority—even those whose depression is extremely severe—can be helped. Thanks to years of fruitful research, there are now medications and psychosocial therapies such as cognitive/behavioral, "talk," or interpersonal that eases the pain of depression.

—NIMH Publication No.
00151–2000

The symptoms of depression can include:

- Persistent sad or "empty" mood
- Loss of interest or pleasure in ordinary activities, including sex
- Decreased energy, fatigue, being "slowed down"
- Sleep disturbances (insomnia, early morning waking, or oversleeping)
- Eating disturbances (loss of appetite and weight, or weight gain)
- Difficulty concentrating, remembering, making decisions
- Feelings of hopelessness, pessimism
- Feelings of guilt, worthlessness, helplessness
- Thoughts of death or suicide; suicide attempts
- Irritability
- Excessive crying
- Chronic aches and pains that don't respond to treatment

—The Symptoms of
Depression
National Mental Health
Association (1997)

The National Institute of Mental Health describes three of the most common types of depressive disorders as follows:

Major Unipolar Depression

This is manifested by the following combination of symptoms: Those that interfere with the ability to work, study, sleep, eat and enjoy once pleasurable activities. Such a disabling episode may occur only once but more commonly occurs several times in a lifetime.

Dysthymia

A less severe type of depression, dysthymia involves long-term, chronic symptoms that do not disable, but keep one from functioning well or from feeling good. Many people with dysthymia also experience major depressive episodes at some time in their lives.

Bipolar or Manic Depression

Another type of depression is bipolar depression, also called manic-depressive illness. Not nearly as prevalent as other forms of depressive disorders, bipolar disorder is characterized by cycling mood changes: severe highs (mania) and lows (depression). Sometimes the mood switches are dramatic and rapid, but most often they are gradual. When in the depressed cycle, an individual can have any or all of the symptoms of a depressive disorder. When in the manic cycle, the individual may be overactive, over talkative, and have a great deal of energy.

—The National Institute
of Mental Health, Publ
#0004501

EDITORIAL

My efforts in this book will be limited to major depression and dysthymia as my personal experiences relate to these forms of mental illness. I don't feel qualified to write on manic depressive disorder. Further, beyond giving some limited statistics of mental illness in children and recommending a source for further study, I do not feel qualified to write in this area. I would suggest that anyone interested in this area could contact the National Association of School Psychologists. This organization offers a variety of publications dealing with student depression in a range of school settings. Its web site is (www.naspweb.org).

Also, I don't feel capable to write regarding the elderly who have multiple disabilities or Alzheimer's disease; although I hope some of my suggestions for coping with depression can be helpful to anyone dealing with this illness.

III
Etiology (Causes) of Depression

From all I have learned over many years of study of depression, my description of the causes, is as follows:

> Depression is caused by a genetic disposition, inherited in the genes, especially those in the brain, triggered by physical and/or stress related to environmental factors during life.

Causes of Clinical Depression:

Many things can contribute to clinical depression. For some people, a number of factors seem to be involved, while for others a single factor can cause the illness. Oftentimes, people become depressed for no apparent reason.

- **Biological**—People with depression typically have too little or too much of certain brain chemicals, called "neurotransmitters." Changes in these brain chemicals may cause or contribute to clinical depression.
- **Cognitive**—People with negative thinking patterns and low self-esteem are more likely to develop clinical depression.

- **Gender**—Women experience clinical depression at a rate that is nearly twice that of men. While the reasons for this are still unclear, they may include the hormonal changes women go through during menstruation, pregnancy, childbirth and menopause. Other reasons may include the stress caused by multiple responsibilities that women have.
- **Co-occurrence**—Clinical depression is more likely to occur along with certain illnesses, such as heart disease, cancer, Parkinson's disease, diabetes, Alzheimer's disease and hormonal disorders.
- **Medications**—Side effects of some medications can bring about depression.
- **Genetic**—A family history of clinical depression increases the risk for developing the illness.
- **Situational**—Difficult life events, including divorce, financial problems or the death of a loved one can contribute to clinical depression.

For additional resources call 1-800-969-NMHA for the National Mental Health Association.

In a recent article, Nancy C. Andreasen, M.D., Ph.D. discusses the latest scientific advances related to the causes of depression. The article is entitled "A Golden Age of Neuroscience." (Nancy C. Andreasen, 2000) discusses latest scientific advances:

We are living in a "golden age" of neuroscience, a time when tremendous discoveries are taking place and will continue to occur. That's the view of one of the world's leading researchers in brain science, Nancy Andreasen, M.D., Ph.D. On the occasion of NARSAD'S Annual Klerman and Freedman Awards ceremony in July, Dr. Andreasen presented a fascinating discussion of research advances.

She took time out from her busy schedule as professor of psychiatry at The University of Iowa College of Medicine, director of The MIND Institute in Albuquerque, NM, and editor-in-chef of *The American Journal of Psychiatry* to discuss two of the most exciting areas of brain research today: Neuroimaging and genetics. A member of NARSAD's Scientific Council, Dr. Andreasen has devoted much of her career to helping to solve the mysteries of schizophrenia (and other forms of mental illness.) She was honored with both the prestigious National Medal of Science and NARSAD'S Lieber Prize in 2000. Her latest book, *Brave New Brain: Conquering Mental Illness in the Era of the Genome,* offers an insider's look at what is known about the human brain.

A pioneer in the development and refinement of many of the neuroimaging tools used in psychiatric research today, Dr. Andreasen noted that two huge domains of knowledge are converging and will lead to tremendous advances in how we understand the normal brain and how we understand mental illness.

> "These two domains of knowledge are at what we call the systems level—areas of cognitive neuroscience, understanding normal behavior and pathological behavior and illnesses, and then at the level of the gene, or the molecular level," she said. "Those two are converging and the process is going to produce an explosion of knowledge and, I believe, tremendous progress in understanding the mechanisms of mental illness and better treatments."

Neuroimaging, which includes CT scanning, PET scanning and magnetic resonance imaging, has become a major scientific domain. "The field has just exploded," she said. "We can literally look inside peoples' heads, look at brain structure, look at brain blood flow, look at chemistry, look at receptors, and neural development."

Dr. Andreasen noted that scientists have begun to recognize schizophrenia (and other forms of mental illness) as a neurodevelopment disorder, and some of the evidence comes from brain imaging studies. "With the tools of functional imaging, we are able to visualize how different regions of the brain, different neural networks, are communicating with one another in an inefficient or inaccurate way, leading to the symptoms that we see, whether delusions, hallucinations or confused thinking."

Using slides to illustrate her point, Dr. Andreasen demonstrated that people with schizophrenia are not activating the same networks of brain regions as healthy controls when performing a task such as working memory. Imaging tests, such as functional MRI, are allowing researchers to identify brain regions that may be impaired.

Imaging tools are also being used to develop a more scientific basis for medication dosing. Using radioactive tracers, researchers can actually see where a drug goes in the brain and how it affects specific brain receptors. Imaging research is beginning to change clinical practice, according to Dr. Andreasen, because it has shown investigators that they can potentially use much lower doses of drugs than traditionally prescribed to achieve the therapeutic effect.

> "We are gradually, steadily building a scientific basis for knowing what doses of drugs to use for our patients to get it exactly right—not too much and not too little. And that's big progress," she said.

Along with brain imaging, Dr. Andreasen noted that

genetics and molecular psychiatry represent the other very exciting frontier in modern psychiatry and neuroscience.

Although the human genome has been decoded, Dr. Andreasen said scientists still have a long way to go in finding better treatments and ways to prevent brain-based illnesses. "They're complex illnesses," she said. "They are not going to be single-gene illnesses. They are going to have two, three, four, five, ten, fifteen or more genes that are interacting with one another. So finding a gene that may play a role in schizophrenia, bipolar illness (Ed. and other forms of mental illness) isn't going to solve the problem totally." Once a gene is found, researchers must get to work on cloning, sequencing, and identifying its products and functions. Even if genes are identified, the role of the environment in illness causation is still very important, she said.

A field known as behavioral neurogenics integrates tools such as brain imaging and genetics, genomics and proteomics. Proteomics is the study of all the proteins produced by cell type and organism.

> "The idea is to look at links between variations in gene alleles and variations in normal functions, or in disease process," she said.
>
> "And this is a really powerful tool for identifying disease vulnerability and the development of treatment."

For example, Daniel Weinberger, M.D., who is on NARSAD's Scientific Council and at the NIMH, found variations in the COMT gene, which is related to dopamine activity in the brain. He showed that variations in this gene affected cognitive function when people performed certain tasks, such as a card-sorting test.

Interestingly, tests such as *f* MRI which measures

blood flow in the brain can also show what is happening in the brain when people perform a mental activity. And the *f* MRI images vary, depending on their particular COMT gene variation.

Dr. Andeasen predicted tremendous discoveries about the mechanisms of mental illness over the next ten to twenty years, in addition to improved treatments and a better understanding of how to prevent some illnesses.

Still, she ended her discussion with a note of caution. While we reap the benefits of new technologies, we must not lose sight of the perils. In the field of genetic testing, for example, how much should people know about their susceptibility for a disease? How much would they want to know? Could insurance companies deny coverage to people at risk for certain illnesses?

She also questions whether the growth in biomedical technology could dehumanize psychiatry. "Increasingly, psychiatrists are being asked to prescribe medications and talk to their patients less. This is being dictated by managed care, HMOs," she said. "That's a terrible loss and I think it's something we'll all have to fight."

She said her guiding framework as a scientist is based on the view held by Albert Einstein. He believed that concern for humankind and our fate must always be the chief interest of all technical endeavors, so that the creations of our mind shall be a blessing, and not a curse, to humanity.

—Nancy Andreasen,
M.D., Ph.D., 2000
(See Bibliography)

EDITORIAL

As one can readily see science has proven that severe mental illness is caused by biochemical imbalance, as well as environmental causes. Years ago, the widely promulgated Freudian concept put the cause strictly on environmental factors, especially on the early life experiences of a person within a dysfunctional family. This caused great trauma to parents. It was due to the stigma they endured resulting from the acceptance and promulgation of this theory, by professionals and the general public. Mental illness is now often referred to as a "no blame disease" although human errors in parenting can be part of the environmental cause of depression.

Another explanation of the causes of depression is given as follows:

Many factors can cause depression, including biochemistry (a chemical imbalance of mood regulation in the brain), genetics, family history, substance abuse, and an illness or other difficult life events. Some people have mild depression, while in others depression is more severe.

—Families for Depression Awareness

IV

Sample Feelings and Actions of Depressed Persons

One day, U.S. President Abraham Lincoln sat down and wrote to his law partner John Stuart: "I am the most miserable man living. If what I feel were equally distributed to the whole human family, there would not be one cheerful face on earth. Whether I shall ever be better, I cannot tell: I awfully forebode I shall not. To remain as I am is impossible. I must die to be better. . . ."

—Judy Falkenberg (1983)
(See Bibliography)

Melancholy and the Muse

Depression seems to be an occupational hazard of many writers and other artists.

Novelist Virginia Woolf and poets Ann Sexton, Sylvia Plath, and John Berryman all committed suicide after bouts with depression. Robert Lowell has written movingly of his depression and repeated hospitalizations.

Nor have musicians been immune to its ravages. Schumann wrote much of his piano music while depressed. He died in an asylum after an earlier attempt at suicide by drowning. Handel wrote his *Messiah* in less than a month during one of his manic or high states.

Whether or not writers had depression, they examined and wrote poignantly of the disorder that so dominates the lives it takes over.

Robert Burton, a seventeenth-century philosopher and humorist, wrote, "All my griefs to this are jolly/naught so damn'd as melancholy." The poet Milton described depression as "demonic frenzy," "moping melancholy," and "moon-struck madness." Shakespeare wrote of "the sad companion, dull-eyed melancholy."

F. Scott Fitzgerald, whose wife was institutionalized for mental illness, and who himself was an alcoholic, evokes the mood of depression in his essay *The Crack-Up* (copyright ©1945 by New Direction Publishing Co.):

> But after three o'clock in the morning, a forgotten package has the same tragic importance as a death sentence, and the cure doesn't work—and in a real dark night of the soul it is always three o'clock in the morning, day after day.

In the novel, *The Sorrows of Young Werther,* the writer Goethe has his character speak in words reminiscent of modern-day patients who describe their depression:

"God knows, I often get into bed with the desire, indeed at times with the hope, of not awaking again, and in the morning I open my eyes, see the sun again, and am wretched. O that I could be capricious, could put the blame on the weather, or a third party, on a frustrated undertaking, then I would only have to bear half the unendurable burden of ill humor. But woe is me! I feel too plainly that all the guilt is mine alone,—no not guilt! Bad enough that in me the source of all my misery lies concealed, as formerly the source of all my joys. . . . My eyes are dried up, and my thoughts, no longer regaled with refreshing tears, draw my brow into anxious folds. I suffer much, for I have lost what was the sole rapture of my life, that holy, animating force with which I created worlds all about me; it is gone!"

—Judy Falkenberg (1983)
(See Bibliography)

Pittsburgh's "Man of Steel," Terry Bradshaw, fifty-five, the Hall of Fame quarterback who later won two Emmys for sports broadcasting recently stated, "I started having breakdowns in my twenties. I tried to make myself happy by winning more games, accumulating more stuff, going through one wife, two wives, three wives. The only thing I could do was work and I worked myself to death, so I could escape." Six years ago Bradshaw learned the reason for the misery that had plagued him for decades: clinical depression.

—Diane Hales, *Parade* Magazine, 2004

Conclusion

My first experience with the feelings and actions related to a clinical depression was at age 50 (1970) as I explained in Chapter I. At this time, I met with my most trusted family doctor. I told him how I felt as a result of my past and present feelings and actions. He was convinced that I needed both medication and psychotherapy and recommended I see a psychiatrist. I will always remember his realistic, yet encouraging words, when he said, "You don't think you'll get better, but you will." I put much faith in his words.

My feelings and actions during this first depression were much more difficult and intense than in my subsequent three episodes leading to the present time (2004). The medication was not nearly as advanced in 1970 and the negative side effects were more pronounced. Also, my coping mechanisms were limited and my fear and the personal stigma I felt, generated from the thought of being mentally ill was greater. I had much trouble sleeping, concentrating, making decisions and staying positive about my present and future life. The thought of taking my life entered my mind, but never became prominent. The love I shared with my wife and family trumped these thoughts, along with my faith in God, friends, and doctors. I imagined I could do some form of work to justify my existence, as long as my dear wife and family could accept my condition.

In my subsequent three depressions in 1983, 1989, and 2001–2002, Prozac became available, which was more helpful in alleviating my depression and it had less negative side effects. In 1983 I retired seven years earlier than required from Springfield College. I had mixed feelings about this decision because I loved my work, as a professor of health and physical education. My love for this college was deep, after thirty-seven years of service there as a teacher and coach. However, my wife Ann had been diagnosed with breast cancer, had endured a radical mastectomy in 1979, and had retired from teaching in her public school position. My retirement would allow us more time together and to follow her condition closely. It worked out that she was allowed twenty years of good living before the cancer reoccurred in 1999. From that point till her death from this disease in December 2001 she lived with great courage and ability to share her love and life with me and many others in this world. For more than three years she endured many treatments with many forms of hormones and chemotherapy. She also took part in a test trial at Boston's Dana Farber Clinic.

In 1983 when I retired I felt feelings of my depression returning. My family doctor had warned me to get on medication and therapy immediately if this happened. I followed his advice and the psychiatrist that I chose said to me, "This depression will not be as difficult as the first because you've been down this road before." Although it was not easy, it was six months before I saw joy again. He was correct. Much of this was the result of my better acceptance of my condition my faith that I would find joy again, and the improved medication.

These episodes and the following two described in Chapter I, bring me to the time when I have gone off all medication for six months in 2003. I have only met for psychotherapy with my psychiatrist once in the past seven months. I can't say I will ever get over the loneliness felt by the loss of my dear wife who was my best friend for nearly sixty-three years, and the one I shared great love with in marriage for just short of sixty years. I do know that she let me know that she wants me to make the most of each day in sharing my love with the God we both loved and the world at large. I'm hoping that I will be reunited with Ann in spite of the mystery of the afterlife. I'm betting my life on it.

Now, in May of 2005, I am on 15 mg. of an antidepressant, Remeron, at bedtime. This is the average level prescribed.

Though it may be only an aspiration in any person's life to live always in a state of high level wellness, I believe that my life has much joy to offer me and I hope to others.

Finally, I must state that I had the great privilege of experiencing a near perfect childhood. I was a most wanted first son in a happy marriage. My mother and father gave me great love and security in my first seven-and-one-half years of life, before my father's death at that time. These most important years in forming one's trust in life have been some great part, in my opinion, in helping as an inoculation, to any long lasting depression. It has aided in my ability to find joy through most of my life. Many persons with depressive illness may not have had this blessing early in life, and I hope this book may help them.

V

My Suggestions for Living with Depression and Finding Joy

1. Physical and Mental Exam and Treatment with Medication and Psychotherapy
2. Gain Love Relationships
3. Stay in the Mainstream
4. Exercise Daily
5. Rest Often
6. The Courage to Be
7. Live for Possibilities
8. Good Nutrition
9. Patience and Faith
10. Prayer
11. Find Reasons to Laugh
12. Be Creative
13. Feel Your Pain. Cry When Appropriate—One Must Go Through It to Get Out of It
14. Help Others in Need—Be Generous—Do Good When No One Is Looking
15. Exchange Smiles and Greetings with People
16. Live with Ambiguity—Accept Yourself and Mystery in Life
17. Belly Breathing—Biofeedback—Relaxation Exercises

18. Evaluate Your Values, From Time to Time, and Live Them
19. Treat Yourself
20. Arrange For a Change of Scenery, Day Trips, Walks or New Experiences
21. Keep Up Your Physical Appearance—Clean, Neat
22. Be Grateful for Blessings, Especially Those Taken for Granted
23. Eliminate Illegal Drugs and Limit or Eliminate Legal Drugs Not Necessary to Treat Illness
24. Light Therapy
25. Utilize the Resources of the National Alliance for the Mentally Ill

One

Physical and Mental Exam and Treatment with Medication, Psychotherapy

I have found that a vital starting point toward reaching the goal expressed in this chapter heading is obtaining high quality professional medical and psychological help. I suggest that one initially get a complete physical exam. This is done to identify any physical cause that can be alleviated with treatment by or other than anti-depressant treatment. Once this physical exam is completed, or even as a physical ailment is being remedied, then I suggest that one needs to have a complete dialogue with a medical doctor, or a psychology professional, qualified to diagnose any mental problem. This should include a lengthy dialogue between the patient and the professional, covering the patient's life history as it could relate to her/his mental condition.

Once the physical and mental picture is complete and a diagnosis is established medication may be recommended by a doctor. If this is the case, I suggest one should follow this recommendation, unless the patient feels the need for a second opinion. There should always be, early and often, follow-up meetings with the chosen doctor, to discuss and evaluate the reaction the patient has to the medication, as time goes by. The medication may have to be changed, either the type or quantity, for best results. With most, if not all medication, it will take some time for the medication to bring the desired results.

Psychotherapy is recommended, starting as soon as the diagnosis indicates that the patient needs treatment for depression.

> The National Institute of Mental Health states, "Yes, depression is treatable. Between 80 and 90 percent of people with depression—even with the most serious forms can be helped."

There are a variety of antidepressants and medications and psychotherapies that can be used to treat depressive disorders. Some people with milder forms may do well with psychotherapy alone. People with moderate to severe depression most often benefit from anti-depressant medications. Most do best with combined treatments: medication to gain relatively quick relief and psychotherapy to learn more effective ways to deal with life's problems, including depression.

"The most important step toward overcoming depression and sometimes the most difficult is asking for help."

—What to Do When a
Friend Is Depressed
National Institute of
Mental Health 12/6/03

The United States Food and Drug Administration (FDA), in the Springfield, Massachusetts *Republican* Newspaper, 8/21/04, states, "We are preparing stronger warnings for some anti-depressants used by children, after new analysis backs a possible link to suicide. Exactly what those warnings will say hasn't been settled according to FDA released Friday. The agency will ask its scientific advisors next month to help in deciding."

(Editorial: It would seem highly advisable for any parents to follow the upcoming evidence on this, through a competent psychological professional, before deciding on the use of antidepressant medication for a child.)

Electroconvulsive Therapy

NMHA supports the position that potential ECT recipients and their significant others, and families or guardians when appropriate, must have access to information on the procedure from a range of sources, both pro and con, to enable them to make truly informed decision about it. Most important, anyone who chooses ECT must do so competently and without coercion.

NMHA recommends that ECT be presented as an alternative with extreme caution, only after all other treatment approaches, such as medication and psychotherapy, have either failed or have been seriously and thoroughly evaluated and rejected.

ECT and the ECT debate have undergone a complete image makeover in the last twenty years. It has regained respectability. Many psychiatrists now consider it an efficient way to relieve severe depression or to break a manic cycle for the manic depressive. Its success rate, according to the American Psychiatric Association (APA), is 80 percent, considerably higher than the 50 percent to 60 percent success rate of most antidepressant medications. And according to ECT advocates, it can restore a severely depressed or manic patient to health in half the time it takes medication—sometimes as little as three weeks to reach a therapeutic level. ECT has made a big comeback and is thought to be kinder and gentler today.

Today ECT is administered to an estimated 100,000 people a year, primarily in general hospital psychiatric units and in psychiatric hospitals. It is generally used in treating patients with severe depression, acute mania, and certain schizophrenic syndromes. ECT is also used with some suicidal patients, who cannot wait for antidepressant medication to take effect.

The patient and physician should discuss all options available before deciding on any treatment. If ECT is recommended, the patient should be given a complete medical examination including a history, physical, neurological examination, EKG, and laboratory test. Medications need to be noted and monitored closely, as should cardiac conditions and hypertension. The patient and family should be educated and informed about the procedure via videos, written material, discussion, and any other means available before a written consent is signed. The procedure should be administered by trained health professionals with experience in ECT administration as well as a specifically trained and certified anesthesiologist to administer the anesthesia. The seizure initiated by the electrical stimulus varies from person to person and should be monitored carefully by the administration team. Monitoring should be done by an EEG or "cuff" technique. The nature of ECT, its history of abuse, unfavorable medical and media reports and testimony from former patients all contribute to the debate surrounding its use. Research should continue, and techniques should be refined to maximize the efficacy and minimize the risks and side effects resulting from ECT. For information contact one of the following sources:

National Mental Health Association
2001 N. Beauregard Street
12th Floor
Alexandria, VA 22311
Phone 800-969-6642
www.nmha.org

National Institute of Mental Health
Public Inquiries
6001 Executive Boulevard
Room 8184, MSC 9663
Bethesda, MD 20892
www.nimh.nih.gov

American Psychiatric Association
1000 Wilson Blvd.
Suite 1825
Arlington, VA 22209
www.psych.org

The following sections are taken from an article posted by Dr. D.J. Jaffe, on the use of ECT in depression, by Dr. Demitris Popolus of Montefiore Medical Center.

ECT Therapy has received some bad press as a result of what the treatment used to be. Yet "ECT has a higher success rate for severe depression than any other form of treatment." It has also been shown to be an effective form of treatment for schizophrenia accompanied by catatonia, extreme depression, mania or other affective components.

ECT has a higher success rate for severe depression than any other form of treatment. It can be life-saving and produce dramatic results. It is particularly useful for people who suffer from psychotic depressions or intractable mania, people who cannot take antidepressants due to problems of health or lack of response and pregnant women who suffer from depression or mania. A patient who is very intent on suicide, and who would not wait three weeks for an antidepressant to work, would be a good candidate for ECT because it works more rapidly. In fact suicide attempts are relatively rare after ECT.

ECT is usually given three times a week. A patient may require as few as three or four treatments or as many as twelve to fifteen. Once the family and patient consider that the patient is more or less back to their normal level of functioning, it is usual for the patient to have one to two additional treatments in order to prevent relapse. Today the method is painless, and with modifications in technique it bears little relationship to the unmodified treatments of the 1940s.

Doctors often underplay the potential side-effects. In addition, it is sometimes prescribed for conditions it is not medically appropriate for. And like other treatments, the effect is not always permanent. Like with medicines, ECT is not used once and you are better forever. Maintenance ECT may be required.

The official policy of the National Alliance for the Mentally Ill (NAMI) is that while it does not endorse particular forms of treatment it believes informed individuals with neurobiological disorders have the right to receive

National Institute of Mental Health approved treatments like ECT from properly trained practitioners. NAMI opposes actions intended to limit this right.

Two

Gain Close Personal Relationships

I have found it most helpful to seek out and establish strong close relationships with many persons in my life. As I explained previously, my family of origin, though truncated by the early deaths of my father and brother, was a great help to me. I also shared much love with my extended family of origin, which was important, especially following the deaths in my family of origin. I have also benefited from the sharing of love with many wonderful friends.

At this point in our discussion of authentic love, I want to tell you about my family by marriage. This family is composed of my wife Ann, daughter Cathy, grandson Matt and son-in-law, Bob Sullivan. They have been vital to my overall well-being during the sun and shadows of my life.

Ann's parents had eloped from Lithuania in about 1900 due to the fact that her father was about to be forcibly conscripted into the Russian army. They worked their way to America where Ann's father, Ignatius, found work in the Pittston, Pennsylvania area, working in the coal mines for ten years. Six children were born to their family in those years.

In 1914 they were able to fulfill a dream when they purchased a farm in central New York State near Hamilton. Subsequently they sold this farm and bought a large dairy farm within two miles of Hamilton. During the years on these farms, three more children were added, Jewel, Ann, and Martha, resulting in a total of nine children; three hardworking, devoted brothers and the "six-pack" of outstanding and beautiful daughters. Most everyone in the Hamilton area knew of the Mordus family and girls, as they were very popular with everyone. Frances started a highly successful hair-dressing business with her partner Alice in 1925. Ann and the other sisters visited her regularly to earn some extra money cleaning the shop and running errands. One time after I became friends with Ann, a kindly Irishman in town, Ward Walsh, who had the gift of blarney, exclaimed, "Ann, you're the flower of the flock." We still accept this as a great compliment, even though we later learned the he told some of the other sisters the same story.

Everyone in Ann's family was highly intelligent. Two sisters were valedictorians of their high school classes. Ann went off to college at the University of the State of New York at Cortland at age fifteen, after having earlier skipped two grades in her one-room elementary school. One teacher taught all eight grades in the school that had about twelve children. To graduate from high school, one had to pass the New York State Regents examinations. When Ann finished the elementary school, she entered Sherburne High School. She worked for her room and board. She lived with a family, as there was no transportation and the family farm was seven miles away from the village. When the family moved to the second farm (Red Gate Stock Farm), it was close enough to the village of Earlville for her to commute to school by bus. Both Sherburne and Earlville are close to Hamilton. Ann became active in sports in Earlville High School both in basketball and track.

There are two stories that Ann loves to tell of her experience in her freshman year at Sherburne High School. As stated previously, at the age of eleven, she worked for her room and board with a very nice family named Nelson. Her duties included being a sitter for their two girls aged four and six, along with helping with dishes and running errands. One day Mrs. Nelson asked Ann to go to the butcher for a half pound of liverwurst, which was an unfamiliar word for Ann. She repeated it to herself all the way to the store, as she has always been extremely conscientious in her duties. When she faced the butcher, her mind did a trick on her and all that came out was, "I want a half pound of worsted liver." Fortunately the butcher said, "I think you mean a half pound of liverwurst." To which Ann replied, "Liverwurst or worsted liver, what is the difference?"

Another time she had the great thrill of finding three one-dollar bills rolled up in a tight roll just outside the Nelsons' on the way to school. She was so excited that she ran all the way to school to tell her sister Jewel, who was a sophomore at Shelburne High School. Jewel was living with another family in town while in high school. Upon meeting Jewel said "last night I came to visit you, I had three dollars—I've lost it." Ann's excitement was dampened for an instant, but soon they were both smiling as Ann saw Jewel so happy now that the lost was found. The Mordus family has always been a very close supportive family, helping each other in time of need and getting together for family fun reunions nearly every year since World War II ended.

When Ann went to the University of New York at Cortland at age fifteen, she had twelve dollars that she had saved working for Frances in her beauty parlor. She hitchhiked a ride to Hamilton with her suitcase in hand from the farm, and from there Fran and her husband Bill Moten gave her a ride to Cortland. She had convinced the admissions director in an earlier interview that she was not too young to make it through Cortland and that she was determined to do it rather than spend the rest of her life helping on the farm. She spent three of the twelve dollars for a room in a tourist home the first night of arrival. The very next day, she found a very nice family named Kelly with whom she could work for her room and board. Mrs. Kelly was a librarian in a neighboring town, and Mr. Kelly was a salesman who traveled a great deal. They had twins in grade school. Ann's job with this family was to be there to supervise the children when they arrived home from school and to assist with the housework. There were no set hours for Ann to clean house. One day Mrs. Kelly evaluated Ann's work by running her finger on the ledge over a door. When she found that Ann had even dusted there, she said, "I'll leave the cleaning up to you to do at your own pace, whenever you find the time. I know you will do a good job."

Her parents gave her some help with money for second-hand books and the physical education uniforms she was able to purchase from a student who decided not to continue in that field. The tuition was only about ten dollars a semester since those were Depression days. Her parents and sister Frances helped her with these expenses. She had good nutritious food for her first two years as she was living with the Kelly family. The final two years she joined four other students in an apartment. She was able to get a job making about two-dollars and fifty cents a week (thirty-three cents per hour) in the college office of Dr. Brown. This was enough to take care of her share of the rent and buy some food. This job was provided by the National Recovery Act under President Franklin Roosevelt. Though it was adequate, she admits she did not always have a good balanced diet during those two final years. After vacations spent at home, she brought food from there (mostly vegetables) to supplement the supply for their apartment.

Because Ann had graduated from college at such a young age, she was ahead of me in schooling. I was still at Colgate when she came home to visit her family on Red Gate Stock Farm. When I went there to visit her, she might be out on the tractor helping her family. I got down to help her and the family take the corn into the silo, as a small contribution to the everlasting work that is needed on a farm. I must admit I was a bit embarrassed one day when we met her father coming out to do very early morning milking chores when we were returning from a long evening date together. He had considerable trust in his six daughters due to the family's great love and attention to each other. Ann was the next to the youngest of nine children, so she had a fine example from her parents, four older sisters and three older brothers.

As a result of Ann's early life experiences in helping with multiple chores on the farm, her work habits surpass mine. By her example she has influenced me to try to upgrade my work habits. Further, she has been a most positive influence on our daughter, Cathy who has achieved a doctorate in educational psychology and has served many years in the Simsbury, Connecticut public schools as a school psychologist.

Ann's most important influence on me has been to help me learn more about the meaning of authentic love. In my early years, I lived to a large extent for the comfort and pleasure of the day, without sufficient concerns for others. I do believe I have learned to act in a more caring way toward others through her example, and I feel good about this. Erik Erikson, a noted psychoanalyst, in his most perceptive theory regarding the psychosocial stages of life, states that the final life stage is a conflict between integrity and despair. Many of us probably have some of each of these feelings, but I sense enough of the positive features of my life at this point, to feel a healthy sense of integrity. Webster's New Collegiate Dictionary (1973) defines integrity as "a firm adherence to a code of moral values."

It took three years of marriage before Ann and I were successful in our desire to have children. During these early years, I was in World War II military service for thirty-nine months. Ann became pregnant with Cathy, our daughter, shortly before my discharge from the Army Air Corps. It was a challenging time, because Ann had given up teaching and we had little money.

However, Ann was most supportive of a plan for me to return to school in pursuit of a Master's Degree in Physical Education at Springfield College, Springfield, Massachusetts. Fortunately we had the G.I. Bill of Rights. Cathy, our wonderful daughter, was born during this school year as we lived in a veterans' housing project. She was born prematurely at seven and one-half months. The doctor told me soon after her delivery, "I think she will live." I headed for the nearest church and prayed, as I never had before, for her healthy survival and development. I don't think I was ever the same person again after her birth and the positive answer to these fervent prayers. Of course, it was Ann's love and courage that made a big difference. She immediately started nursing and nurturing Cathy, and she thrived on it, gaining weight quickly along with overall health. Cathy was to be our only child, even though we worked with an outstanding doctor in a long-term regimen designed to enhance the possibility of pregnancy. There were no fertility drugs at that time. We did look into adoption but perhaps became too easily discouraged by the long time frame and other hurdles to overcome.

I received a master's degree at Springfield College in

1947 and a most fortunate appointment to the faculty of Springfield College. We decided that Ann should be a mother and housewife for the early years of Cathy's development. We bought a brand new Cape Cod-style home on a G.I. loan for $7,700 and were a happy family. I had a good summer job as a recreation director at Longmeadow, Massachusetts, a suburb of Springfield. This job paid $1,000 to supplement the $2,700 I earned for the nine months on the Springfield college faculty. This was six years after our wedding. We had very little money saved, but we felt pretty secure and fortunate to have found our niche in life. We had grown up during Depression days and we were not used to many luxuries, even though we knew that many were more economically troubled than our family at that time. After Ann went back to teaching when Cathy reached junior high school, we started our own business together. It was a day camp called Camp Husky, open to girls and boys aged five to eleven for ten weeks in the summer. We operated this business for fourteen years, before terminating it in 1967. It was thriving at that point, but we wanted a bit of time in the summer to enjoy ourselves. Cathy had helped us immensely with the camp as a junior and senior counselor, and she was graduating from Skidmore College and getting married in August 1968 to Bob Sullivan, a former "best camper" at Camp Husky.

We have some great memories of the children who attended our camp. Ann and I always referred to each other in front of the campers as Mrs. and Mr. Dunn. Occasionally we would call across the campgrounds to each other using the first names Ann and Ted. One of the young boys came up to Ann one day and said, "How come you call him Ted and he calls you Ann, how come?"

One of our sharp five-year-olds, a long-term summer camper, was the son of a prominent doctor. He had an older brother and sister who also attended camp, so he tried to keep up with them. He always wanted to be left off last when I took a group of campers home at day's end. For several days I was able to pacify Johnnie by saying, "We'll see, Johnnie." He might then often fall asleep the rest of the way to his home. He wasn't too happy when he wasn't left off last, however. One day, when I gave him the "we'll see" response, he stated flatly, "I've had enough of the 'we'll see,' I want an answer yes or no." Perhaps he had read the quote of St. Augustine, "By and by never comes."

One of our main objectives at camp was to teach each child to reach a reasonably high level of skill in swimming. We had two pools—a beginner pool above ground and an advanced deep-water concrete pool. Many of the five-year-olds could not swim on arrival, although some would say, "I used to know how to swim, but I forgot how." Ann took the greatest pride in teaching beginners and she was as thrilled as they were when they gained confidence in learning to swim. The thousands of children both at camp and in public school junior high, whom she taught to swim, could alone gain her a slot in heaven.

So Ann and I were a pretty good team for nearly sixty years of marriage. Our experience ranges from living in a one-room apartment with kitchen and bathroom shared with other army personnel (and cockroaches as well) in San Antonio, Texas, in World War II days to our new $7,700 home in 1947, to our recent years of active comfortable retirement in our present home.

I am sure that my life has been much better because Ann has been willing to share it with me. Yes, like most every couple, we have had our times of anger and disagreement. I must admit that my selfishness has been the root of much of this. But each time that happened, we have been willing to start again and build on the good in our relationship. James Thurber, a great American humorist, has quoted a woman who had been married twenty-six years with six children as follows: "Love is something you've been through with someone." This may be one of the best reasons for staying the course in shared love, to reach the promised land of authentic love. As a result of her breast cancer, in December, 2001 we had to ask for the great help of Hospice and Ann died at home on December 29. She taught me by her actions how to live and die. I hope I can follow her example.

I hope readers can appreciate how much Ann has helped me through my depressions. I trust you can appreciate after reading about Ann's many positive qualities, why I have told our daughter in that popular phrase, "I had one-hundred wives, but they were all your mother." Following her death I experienced my longest depressive episode and was on Prozac again for eighteen months, along with regular sessions with a psychiatrist. I also benefited from many free of charge church, hospital, hospice and American Cancer Society supportive groups. I can only hope that others with depression can find great love to share with others in their lives, as I have shared with family and friends.

In addition to human relationships many persons, including myself, have benefited from animal relationships (in my case three different dogs). This form of relationship has been used successfully in assisted living facilities and may be helpful for anyone with a depressive illness.

As stated earlier close personal relationships are vital in the life of a person who is living with depression and hoping to find joy. The following verse by Dinah M. Crack describes this important point.

Friendship

Oh the comfort—the inexpressible
Comfort of feeling safe with a person,
Having neither to weigh thoughts
Nor measure words—but pouring them
All right out—just as they are
Chaff and grain together
Certain that a faithful hand will
Take and sift them
Keep what is worth keeping
And with the breath of kindness
Blow the rest away.

Three

Stay in the Mainstream

I have found it beneficial to stay in the mainstream of life, rather than going in the hospital, when I am depressed. There may be cases where hospitalization is appropriate, especially when there is no family support, or the person cannot function alone. Staying in the mainstream allows one to feel less stigma, sometimes associated with hospitalization, as well as more self sufficient and confident in their ability to get well. This can be true even though one needs to limit their activities, due to less energy during their illness. Fortunately, the stigma is much less today, than in the past, as scientific evidence proves that depression is significantly caused by an imbalance of brain chemicals. Therefore, it is much like cancer or other physically related illnesses, rather than any weakness of character, as sometimes perceived in the past.

Four

Exercise Daily

Daily exercise has proven to be a great help to me throughout life in maintaining physical, mental and spiritual health. It is especially beneficial when I am in depression and am trying to improve my mental health. In my case I jogged, nearly daily, for many years. At my present condition, following four hip operations, I get most of my exercise walking an extra two to three miles a day, rain, snow or shine. These operations may be related to nine years of high school and college football and a genetic factor, as my father used a cane in walking. It is possible for me to find a convenient place to walk out of doors and still be under cover, at a nearby school, in inclement weather. Walking out of doors at least an hour a day is my regimen. Something tells me that outdoor exercise is best because it provides fresh air and spaciousness. Anyone can usually find these ingredients for their outdoor exercise when they use some ingenuity. Our predecessors in this world lived and worked mostly outdoors. Researchers at Texas A & M University found that people who spend time out of doors have lower blood pressure, less anxiety and feel less pain, than indoor types. Researcher Roger Utrich, Ph.D. states, "Spend just three minutes outside daily to get some benefits." In my case I aim for a minimum of one hour outside, in all seasons, unless there is a real danger. However, some may prefer or find it more feasible to exercise partly or mostly indoors, which is also a good choice for them. Walking stairs is a good exercise, rather than taking the elevator. Floor exercises, as well as aerobic exercises, on my leg and arm machine, for regular intervals indoors at home are also helpful.

Exercise has been proven helpful to persons in depression in several scientific studies as follows:

> Psychiatric researchers in the Department of Psychiatry and Behavioral Sciences at Duke University have completed a breakthrough study comparing the use of exercise versus Zoloft, in order to determine the relative effectiveness (or ineffectiveness) of each approach plus a combined approach in patients diagnosed with major depression. Their study was published in Psychosomatic Medicine (Babyak et al., 2000) and was summarized in the February 2002 issue of *Consumer Reports on Health* (Sandroff, 2002).
>
> In the initial Duke study, which lasted for just four months, 156 patients diagnosed with major depression, were randomly assigned to one of three interventions; exercise, the antidepressant Zoloft, or both. After four months, patients in all three groups showed improvement. However, after ten months, those in the exercise group had significantly lower relapse rates ($p=.01$) than those in the medication group and those in the exercise plus medication group. In fact, depressive symptoms had returned in only 8 percent of the exercise-only patients whose symptoms had initially disappeared. This compares with 38 percent in the drug group and 31 percent in the exercise-plus-drug group. "This finding was an unexpected finding because it was assumed that combining exercise with medication would have, if anything, an additive effect." (p. 636)

German researchers have also found that exercise can work in a very effective way in alleviating symptoms of depression. Their research is reported in the *British Journal of*

Sports Medicine. This journal published a study completed by Dr. Fernando Dimeo of the Freie University of Berlin on the benefits from aerobic exercise in patients with major depression (Dimeo, 2001). Dimeo had his subjects walking on a treadmill for thirty minutes per day. Three minutes of intense activity were alternated with walking at half-speed for three minutes. The intensity was increased as heart rate adapted to the training program. Depression severity was measured at the start and end of the program and subjects rated their mood at the beginning, middle, and end of the ten days using a recognized evaluation scale. After ten days, half of the patients were substantially less depressed, including a number for whom drug treatment had been largely unsuccessful. Overall, depression score fell by one third.

The January 2002 issue of *Discover Magazine* (Glausiusz, 2002) includes a research study completed by biochemist Ellen Billet of Nottingham Tern University in England. Billet began studying the molecule phenylethylamine because earlier studies showed that this molecule can modulate levels of mood-altering serotonin and dopamine in the brain. In her study, she asked "twenty healthy men to refrain from exercise on one day and then run on a treadmill for thirty minutes the next day. She took urine samples from subjects on both days and discovered that the concentrations of phenylacetaic acid, a breakdown product of phenyl ethylamine, increased by an average of 77 percent after exercise." (p. 15) This particular molecule is able to cross from the blood stream to the brain, so it might help mediate the connection between exercise and mood in the body's peripheral tissues. "The molecule is also chemically similar to amphetamine, a hint that it might be one source of runner's high. The latest findings may encourage a more holistic approach to psychiatry." (p. 15)

The American Psychological Association website references additional studies showing many benefits of regular exercise in an article entitled "Exercise Helps Keep Your Psyche Fit." (www.apa.org/releases/exercise.html) The author points out that recent review of psychological research shows that exercise is an effective but underused treatment for mild to moderate depression. There is also evidence to indicate that regular exercise can help in the treatment of other mental health problems including alcohol dependence and anxiety disorders. They conclude that, "Considering the evidence that exercise is a viable, cost-effective treatment for depression and chronic pain, the researchers say that they are somewhat surprised that it does not become a more popular treatment alternative and suggest that it be more commonly used as part of a therapist-structured treatment program." (APA. 199, p.1)

The January 2002 issue of *Consumer Reports on Health* has a valuable article entitled, "What Can You Do to Boost Your Energy Level?" This article references the roles of sleep, medication and nutrition as well as exercise in alleviating depression and improving energy levels. The authors point out that, "Exercise and energy are first cousins, and one of the best ways to increase your sense of energy is to work out moderately (extremely strenuous exercise is tiring, not energizing). As you move from a quiet state to an active one, your whole body shifts into a higher gear. Your metabolism and the transmission of nerve impulses speed up, your cardiovascular system works harder and there are changes in hormone secretion. At a conscious level you feel more energetic following exercise. For more energy, build exercise into your day. Experts recommend thirty minutes of moderate exercise most days of the week, which can be done in small bursts, like briskly walking from the back of the parking lot to the store." (Sandroff, 2002, p.6) They also note that the average person needs seven to eight hours of sleep a night and studies have shown that if you skip a half-hour sleep you are less alert the next day. If you lose an hour of sleep your mental and physical performance is likely to be impaired. The authors also expressed concern that antidepressants such as Prozac, Zoloft, and other SSRI's can cause daytime fatigue because they often disrupt some people's sleep.

Conclusion

An important message from these studies is that exercise can be a very effective way of alleviating depression. In some cases exercise works much more effectively than antidepressants. The judicious use of exercise combined with helping clients to improve sleep habits and move to plant based nutrition (Johnson, 2002) can offer even greater benefits. Consulting and counseling that incorporates these approaches can enhance virtually any individual's decision making and problem solving as he or she tries to alleviate feelings of depression. As psychologists, we should be focusing on helping clients to develop self-understanding and help them become more aware of how to improve sleep habits, nutritional habits, medication practices and exercise practices.

Editorial: Common sense indicates that regular exercise with consideration for calories taken in and calories expended will allow one to keep a healthy weight. This holistic approach is likely to be much more beneficial than encouraging those drug oriented approaches that offer the false promise of "quick fixes" and often include significant and even deadly adverse side effects. Naturally thorough psychological assessments, appropriate medical and nutritional assessments should be part of the intervention process.

References

American Psychological Association (1999). Exercise helps keep your psyche fit: Research shows exercise to be a viable, cost-effective treatment for depression and may be in the treatment of other mental disorders.
http://www.apa.org/releases/exercise.html.

Five

Rest Often

Depression saps one's energy, so adequate rest is necessary. When dealing with depression, I try to keep regular hours for night sleeping. This means usually for me to be in bed by ten P.M. and up by 6:30 A.M. If I have kept a health regimen of nutrition, exercise and other factors expressed herein, I will usually sleep reasonably well at night. This is a great help to me in improving my mental health when depressed and finding joy in life again. A short nap may also help in restoring energy during the day. The former director of physical education at Springfield College, Dr. Ellis Champlin, used to say that he was a "stroke-glide" person. He would do physical or mental effort, requiring work at times each day, the stroke phase, and then take a rest in the glide phase. My old college football coach at Colgate University, Andy Kerr, said something to me one day that I took as a compliment. When I sat down during practice break on a hot day he said "Ted, a good athlete knows when to relax."

In recent studies it seems to indicate that sleep deprivation may be related to depression. The following article appeared in the *Texas Christian University Daily Skiff*, 7/12/2003. The author is Howard Markel of the *New York Times* newspaper. His article states "Like many college students, Jenny Walker, twenty-one is something of a night owl. In her first weeks at the University of Michigan a few years ago, Walker rarely went to bed before three or four A.M."

"In college," she said, "your mom isn't there to tell you to go to bed, and for me, things only got worse. Within a month, I was staying up all night, going to bed at nine A.M. and pretty much missing all my classes. Many nights I would sit with my textbooks, but I couldn't concentrate. I wouldn't let myself get to bed until I finished the work.

"But it was a vicious cycle. The later I stayed up, the worse my concentration got, making studying pretty much impossible. I would read the same paragraphs over and over, and pretty much cried about it."

Three months later, Walker was told that she had clinical depression, and she temporarily withdrew from college.

Her history is not uncommon. In the last few years, mental health professionals have asked whether sleep deprivation plays a role in the increase in cases of depression reported on campuses.

According to a study by psychologists at Kansas State University and published in February in Professional Psychology, the number of college-aged students treated for depression has doubled since 1989. The study involved more than 10,000 students at more than 100 colleges.

The incidence is twice the rate for the general population: One in ten men and one in four women will have a clinical depressive episode in their lifetimes. Since 1989, the number of college students consulting doctors for sleep problems increased even more, some experts say.

"There's no question that college kids are sleeping less than they used to," said Dr. Roseanne Armitage, director of the sleep and Chronophysiology Laboratory at the University of Michigan Depression Center.

Last year, college students averaged 6 to 6.9 hours of sleep a night, far less than the suggested 8 to 9.25 and down from 7 to 7.5 in the 1980s.

Psychiatrists are not certain whether sleep problems are a potential cause or a symptom of depression. Treating depression with anti-depressants is not always as effective for sleep problems as for other symptoms. Some medications like the widely prescribed selective serotonin reuptake inhibitors can actually cause insomnia.

The role of sleep disturbances in depression, however, gained the interest of neuroscientists when a study from the National Institute of Mental Health in 1989 reported that sleep disturbances lasting longer than two weeks increased the risk of developing many psychiatric illnesses, especially depression.

"A good analogy," Dr. Armitage said, "would be having high serum cholesterol and the risk of heart attacks. Just because you have a high cholesterol level does not necessarily mean you are definitely going to have a heart attack. But it is definitely a risk factor. The same could be said for sleep disturbances and the risk of developing depression."

—From *Texas Christian University Daily Skiff*

(Editorial: Part of staying reasonably rested is also involved in keeping a balance in the amount of stress one can afford when depressed. Stressful influences have been categorized into two parts, eustress: that part which is the good stress needed to motivate one to be creative and distress, which is too much stress which can lead to poor health. One needs to limit stressful influences to the amount one can tolerate when depressed, which is normally less than one can when they are well.)

Six

The Courage to Be

The courage to be is a vital force in getting through depression and finding joy. Shakespeare said so clearly in the words "To be or not to be, that is the question." This requires that one chooses to believe that life is worth living and pledges each new day to make it worthwhile in helping oneself and others. William James, a great psychological philosopher, makes this point well when he states "Believe that life is worth living and your belief will create the fact. Be not afraid to live."

Seven

Live For Possibilities

Emily Dickinson, a foremost American poet and a somewhat reclusive individual, lived through a most productive life. This was true though many of her poems were sad and about death. In her difficult moments, she said that she lived for possibilities. My family doctor in consultation during my first depression helped me live for possibilities when he said, "You don't think you'll get better but you will." My psychiatrist during my second episode likewise reminded me, "This depression won't be as difficult as your first because you've been down this road before." I suggest that persons with depression must use all their will, along with creative and positive thinking, to envision better possibilities for today and tomorrow.

A friend of mine likes to use this quote to indicate the importance of keeping hope alive for future good possibilities, "we all need some hope to cling to, some rainbow in the sky."

Eight

Good Nutrition

A nutritious diet is important in coping with and recovering from depression. My suggestion would be to eat a well-balanced diet each day, in this way if possible: A hearty breakfast helps to enter the day following, I hope, a good night's rest. This is followed, where possible, with another hearty meal at noontime. These two meals provide the maximum energy for the most important hours of the day, where it is normally needed. I suggest a more limited supper because normally less energy is needed in the evening hours. If this noon, big meal, isn't possible due to work, then an early dinner in the evening is best.

There are many diets to choose from in the literature. I

prefer the one that is based on a long history of a people from a region of our world around the Mediterranean Sea. It is called "The Mediterranean Diet." It may help you live longer, lower your risk of heart disease and cancer and lower your cholesterol. It also will provide the energy you need and help you keep your weight under control, when followed properly and combined with adequate exercise.

It has been shown by scientific data that those parts of the Mediterranean region where people have enjoyed the lowest recorded rates of chronic diseases and the highest adult life expectancy have a population that continues to eat a diet like the "Mediterranean Diet Health Weight Plan."

Key features of the Mediterranean diet:

- High consumption of breads, pasta, rice, couscous, polenta, bulgur and potatoes
- High consumption of fruits (3–4 pieces a day), legumes and vegetables (5 different varieties)
- Moderate amounts of grilled and steamed fish
- Moderate amounts of olive oil—consumed with fresh vegetables and on salads
- Small portions of lean red meat with no visible fat, lean pork
- Alcohol in small mounts (Editorial: This limits men to no more than two moderate-sized drinks, joined with food, a day and women to no more than one. Some who cannot tolerate alcohol may have to eliminate this part of the diet.)
- High intake of antioxidants
- Regular exercise is believed to be such an important part of Mediterranean health that it is part of the Mediterranean pyramid. This can also aid in maintaining appropriate weight control.

For more information look on the Internet for Mediterranean Diet and the Traditional Healthy Mediterranean Diet Pyramid.

Nine

Patience and Faith

One must learn patience and faith to get through depression and find joy. It has been said that "faith is patience, waiting for a nibble." Faith may be related to one's religious belief in the goodness and the help they will receive from their God and good people. Or it may be their determination to do what is necessary, in doing their duty to be responsible for correcting their condition. There is a faith that somehow when one tries in this life, good results will come. Often, little good feelings, along the way, can be the nibbles that can strengthen one's faith in further successful living. A great priest I knew in the past, emphasized both the religious element in faith as well as the secular, when he said, "Pray as if all depended on God and work as if it all depended on you."

The greatest test of faith, in my estimation, is the question of whether there is a life after death. Many people choose to believe as I do, that this is possible even though it is a mystery, and to my knowledge cannot be proven. In my faith I especially hope to be united with my loved ones. I have sufficient faith in this potential for me, that I join the great seventeenth century French scientific genius, Blaise Pascal, who stated he could not prove the reality of the afterlife but he was "betting his life on it." Robert Browning, one of England's most distinguished nineteenth-century poets, took a stand on this noble test of faith with these memorable lines:

Ah, but a man's reach
Should exceed his grasp,
Or what's a heaven for?

(Editorial: I am sure he used the word man in a generic sense to mean all persons.)

Ten

Prayer

Prayer can be an important part of living with depression and finding joy. *Parade* magazine recently had an excellent article citing considerable research on how prayer and faith speed recovery in illnesses from depression along with stroke and heart attack.

With funding from the National Institutes of Health (NIH), investigators at Johns Hopkins University are studying a group of women with breast cancer who say a meditative prayer twice daily. At the University of Pennsylvania neuroscientists are documenting changes in brain scans of meditating Tibetan Buddhists and praying nuns. At Baptist Memorial Hospital in Memphis, patients are receiving a "prayer intervention" before and after bypass surgery.

"We are not out to prove that a deity exists," says Prof. Diane Becker of Johns Hopkins, recipient of two NIH grants for research on prayer. "We are trying to see whether prayer has meaning to people that translates into biology and affects a disease process."

Medical acceptance has grown along with solid scientific data on prayer's impact, says Dr. Dale Matthews of Georgetown University, author of *The Faith Factor.* He estimates that about 75 percent of studies of spirituality have confirmed health benefits.

Dozens of studies have shown that individuals who pray regularly and attend religious services stay healthier and live longer than those who rarely or never do—even when age, health, habits, demographics and other factors are considered. A six-year Duke University study of 4000 men and women of various faiths, all over age sixty four, found that the relative risk of dying was 46 percent lower for those who frequently attended religious services.

Prayer—whether for oneself (petitionary prayer) or others (intercessory prayer) affects the quality, if not the quantity of life, says Dr Harold Koenig, director of Duke University's Center for the Study of Religion/Spirituality and Health: "It boosts morale, lowers agitation, loneliness and life dissatisfaction, and enhances the ability to cope in men, women, the elderly, the young, the healthy and the sick."

Another Duke study of the same group of 4000 people over sixty four, found that those who prayed regularly had significantly lower blood pressure than the less religious. A third study showed that those who attended religious services had healthier immune systems than those who did not.

—"Why Prayer Could Be
Good Medicine"
Diane Hales
Parade Magazine,
3/23/2004

Eleven

Find Reasons to Laugh

It can be helpful when one is depressed to try to find reasons for laughter, especially laughing at oneself as well as other comedy actions in our many pratfalls. Sometimes, thinking back, humor is tragedy plus time. The University of California Berkeley Health Letter states:

> Laughter reduces tension, clears the mind, and lifts the spirits. The study of humor and its effects on the human body has a name: gelotology. Researchers found laughter improves muscle tone and circulation. Now neurologists at Stanford University have discovered another reason why laughter makes us feel good. They monitored the brain activity of people reading funny cartoons and found that humor and laughter triggered the brain's "reward centers." These are the same areas activated by cocaine and amphetamines. Perhaps this is why laughter is habit forming.

I suggest that one in depression should try to laugh several times each day. It has been said that laughter is the lubrication of life and that laughter is a form of courage.

Twelve

Be Creative

It is important to find something creative to do in getting through depression and finding joy again in life. It is good if this endeavor is something that one can be proud of, because it has some value to others beyond her- or himself. This point is expressed well in the book *Master Game* as follows:

> Seek above all, for a game worth playing. Such is the advice of the oracle to modern man. Having found it play it with intensity—play it as if your life and sanity depended on it. (They do depend on it). Follow the example of the French existentialists and flourish a banner bearing the word, "engagement." Though nothing means anything and all roads are marked "no exit" yet move as if your movements had some purpose. If life does not offer a game worth playing, then invent one.

This may involve some risk of failure, but one can remember the old saying, "When one door closes another may open."

A poem by Sir Walter Scott, in the *Lady of the Lake,* states of the need to take a risk, necessary to be creative, as follows:

> He either fears his fate too much
> Or his deserts are small
> Who dares not put it to the test?
> To gain or lose it all.

(Editorial: As a college teacher of holistic health, I have come to believe that the most important element in seeking high level wellness is, "finding something to be healthy for." Finding something creative, that captures one's devotion, can be a thing that helps one to develop the healthy state needed to be creative. This concept can be applied to many of the other suggestions included in Chapter 5.)

Thirteen

Feel Your Pain, Cry When Appropriate

It can be therapeutic to feel one's pain, at times when one is depressed. These feelings can be vocally expressed to a psychological or medical counselor, in grief groups, and within friends and family. It has been said that one needs to go through depression to get out of it. This may mean recognizing one's feeling openly with words, feelings and tears. It is legitimate to do this at times, as Robert Frost expresses in a poem called "Reluctance," with these words:

> And when to the heart of man
> Was it ever less than treason
> To go with the drift of things
> And yield with a grace to reason
> To bow and accept the end
> Of a love or a season

Naturally one should try to emphasize the positive most of the time when depressed, but it can help also to get our honest feelings expressed in appropriate settings. Also a certain amount of pain felt can cause one to be more grateful for the good times and also more sensitive to the needs of others who are in pain.

Fourteen

Help Others in Need—Be Generous—Do Good When No One Is Looking

In many forms of depression one has feelings of guilt, over past failures of omission in their duties or commission of regrettable acts. These feelings may be alleviated to a degree and replaced by more positive feelings about oneself, by helping others in need of assistance. For conscientious persons the road to personal redemption for past mistakes can be the longest road. Helping others can shorten the road. Even more important is the satisfaction one can derive, in seeing their help shared with other peoples efforts, bring about some good in both their lives.

Fifteen

Exchange Smiles and Greetings with People

It helps me and I hope it would help others in depression to exchange smiles with family and friends and neighbors (Editorial: I use the term neighbors in a broad sense, to include store clerks and others that we meet on a daily basis, in our neighborhood.) Emily Dickinson has a great poem on the value of smiles as follows:

They might not need me
Yet they might,
So I'll keep my heart
Just in sight.
For a smile like mine
Just might be
Precisely their necessity.

This poem indicates a shared value to the extending of smiles. In concert with an exchange of smiles is the good that can come from a shared greeting. I prefer to say, "I hope you have a good day" rather than "Have a good day." This seems a bit like an order rather than a desire expressed from friend to friend, even though this is usually said with good will.

Sixteen

Live with Ambiguity—Accept Yourself and Mystery in Life

Strive to live peacefully with ambiguity in making life's decisions. I have found it difficult at times to make decisions when I'm depressed. Sometimes there are no answers relating to my search for an objective answer for the reality of God. A noted theologian Karl Rahner, in his description is about the best I can find when he states, "God is the incomprehensible mystery, yet everywhere obvious." Examples of more mundane decisions that are difficult are, what medication to take and how much to stretch one's endurance when depressed.

I wrote this poem, "Living," during one of my episodes of depression in 1975.

For nine months my life seemed so good.
The "life of Riley" so they say.
I wished it would never end.
But suddenly that life did end,
or so it seemed,
as out of my mother's womb I was pushed and
    tugged,
into the bright light of day.
It hurt my sensitive eyes and I cried out.
Why did the good life have to end?
Now I understand.
Though never secure,
life in God's earth womb is better still,
with such potential for good,
and bad too, but mostly good,
so challenging—exciting,
so much love abounds, in spite of our
    selfishness
so much joy, in spite of the sadness.
And life became so meaningful
when I first discovered it was far too short
to ever play all the exciting games,
to win and to lose but to play.
What is the answer to this longing to be more
    fully involved,
in all the mysteries that give life meaning?
Perhaps, someday I will know the answer,
when I am pushed and tugged, into the womb
    of God.

The following poem by Maria Rilke has given me comfort when I was dealing with ambiguity.

Be patient with all that is unsolved in your
    heart
Learn to love the questions
Seek not the answers that cannot be given
For you could not live them
Learn to love the questions now
And perhaps in some far distant day
You may live into the answers.

Seventeen

Belly Breathing—Biofeedback—Relaxation Exercises

I first learned of the value of what is commonly called belly breathing at Boston University, where I was working on a doctoral degree in health education in 1980. Since then it has become a vital part of my regimen in trying to relax at all times, especially during moments of stress. Belly breathing is the natural way a baby breathes with its stomach pushing out as they inhale deeply and deflating as they exhale fully. A female nurse recently told me this form of breathing is easier for men, in our society as they more naturally let their stomach extend out as they breathe in whereas women tend to hold their stomachs in when inhaling and inhale with the chest expanding. I don't know whether this is a cultural factor or a biological one, as it relates to women. I strongly believe that women can learn this technique with practice and could benefit from the added vital oxygen it provides to their system, especially during depression.

Eighteen

Evaluate Your Values, From Time to Time, and Live Them

It has been wisely said, that the unexamined life is not worth living. I believe it is helpful for a person in depression to heed this advice and examine the values that they use, to rule their daily actions. A person in depression usually has some good feelings and also some regrets about their past life. An excellent way to build one's self image is to feel one is improving their actions in life. One can accomplish this by examining one's values and the consequences of them in his/her life as well as in the lives of others. As an example of this, I have often used the expression I heard from a black minister, as follows, "I'm not what I could be and I'm not what I should be, but I'm more than I used to be." As one experiences positive changes in their daily actions which please them, they are taking steps out of depression toward joyful living.

Nineteen

Treat Yourself

I believe it is important for a person attempting to move out of depression towards joyful living, to look for ways to treat oneself well. One might examine this concept by using the trick (bad treatment) or treat (good treatment) of the Halloween practice of youngsters. When one is depressed there may be a tendency to practice asceticism, this form of self punishment can be used by the person to alleviate the feelings of guilt or shame one feels for one's condition. In its extreme it may result in an attempt at, or even completion of suicide. My suggestion would be for a person in this state to look for ways to treat themselves well. This can be done by seeking pleasurable activities that are available and are often free of charge. One that immediately comes to mind is to get out walking, enjoying the beauty of nature. A second could be sharing hugs with willing partners. A third could be eating delicious food of many kinds and even some of what my dear departed wife used to call the "morale food group" such as chocolate and other sweets. There are many more treats available to creative persons.

I hope that persons in depression can find joyful living through using some of the activities suggested in this book.

Twenty

Arrange for a Change of Scenery—Day Trips, Walks, or New Experiences

There is a tendency for one in depression to become reclusive. It is expressed by a great author, Nathaniel Hawthorne in these words:

"I have secluded myself from society;
and yet I never meant any such thing.
I have made a captive of myself and put me into
    a dungeon,
And now I cannot find the key to let myself
    out."

Some degree of this desire to be alone when ill may be prudent, in order for one to get some extra rest and lessen their stress level. However, I have found it helpful at times to arrange for a change of scenery in my life when depressed, even though it may be an effort to get up and go. I believe that one will find that once they get out of their home, or restrictive locale, and out for a long walk, a day trip or an overnight visit, they will normally be refreshed. This will often occur because they will open up their world, gain confidence that they can cope with a wider range of people, and this new environment. It may be best to move out from a person's safe haven to a wider world in a gradual way. As one gets more nibbles of joy in their life one can start to extend their horizons. Each time this attempt at becoming part of a wider world is successful, a persons self image and confidence will grow. There may be a setback along the way, but if it is done as suggested here, one will develop joy and confidence, the way one builds a house, brick by brick. Watch how the nibbles of joy increase to become a full size bite of happiness.

Twenty-one

Keep Up Your Physical Appearance—Clean, Neat

My experience with depression has led me to believe it is important for anyone with this illness to keep up their appearance. There can be a temptation to let down one's neat and clean appearance during depression. However, it is even more important for one in this condition to keep their self image, relating to their appearance, at a high level. I'm not referring to any form of high fashion, but just primarily being neat and clean, to a well acceptable degree. This standard of appearance will not only allow the depressed person to feel proud of one self, but will also help others to relate more comfortably with this person.

Twenty-two

Be Grateful for Blessings, Especially Those Taken for Granted

I believe it is helpful for a depressed person to think often about all the things for which they can feel gratitude. There are so many wonderful parts of most anyone's life, that often we take for granted. Some examples are the ability to walk, to talk, to see, to hear, to enjoy good food, to share love and friendship, to pray, to read good literature, view art and listen to good music. This list could be expanded and added to each day when one is creative and is willing to take the time to think about the many things, which are sources of gratitude. I have talked to friends that often take the time to write down a list of things that come to mind, this provides them with a source of gratitude in their lives. This has helped them even during their difficult times.

Twenty-three

Abstain from the Use of Illegal Drugs and Abuse of Legal Drugs

I recall reading a quote from the deceased monk, Baudelaire, who stated, "Every person has a taste for the infinite." To me this means the desire one has to seek a higher level of being than one is accustomed to on earth. This might be sought by a person in depression through the use or abuse of illegal or legal drugs (such as alcohol or tobacco). I would strongly recommend that it is a false lead for anyone with depression to use illegal drugs or abuse legal drugs, especially alcohol and tobacco. Drugs of these types have even led to intentional or unintentional deaths. Mixing these forms of drugs with prescribed medication for mental illness can be dangerous to one's health in many cases. They can also become addictive leading to what is called a "dual diagnosis," which means that a person has a mental illness as well as an addiction to drugs. This results in a double danger to one's health. Jean K. Bouricius in her scholarly books on the topic of psychotoxic drugs, legal and illegal, states, "Fewer than five percent of persons with mental illness were able to continue with moderate drinking, without progressing to alcoholic disorder." Scientific studies have recently shown that alcoholic beverages in moderation can be beneficial to some persons in maintaining heart health. This is recommended in the Mediterranean diet which includes small amounts of red wine with one meal per day. It is further included in the book, *The Healthy Heart,* which recommends, for those who are able to use alcohol in moderation, a maximum of one drink a day with a meal. It warns that any more can raise the blood pressure and increase one's risk of cancer.

Bouricius states that smoking or chewing tobacco is a real danger to one's health and, therefore abstinence is her recommendation, when used in either of these forms. She does note that the nicotine patch or nicotine gum, when used under a doctor's prescription and supervision, may be helpful in the thought process for some persons with mental illness.

> "It has been suggested that nicotine may actually act as an antidepressant in some cases. What is more obvious is that withdrawal from nicotine can precipitate depression. Nicotine might, conceivably, have antidepressant effects resulting from its stimulation of dopamine release. Tricyclic antidepressants, used over a period of time, also augment dopamine release, and thus might be helpful for preventing depression associated with nicotine withdrawal."

Therefore in most cases it seems prudent to rely on antidepressant medication to affect the dopamine release.

Twenty-four

Light Therapy

Another form of therapy that was recommended to me by my psychiatrist is called Light Therapy. I have not used it because I am able to get outside daily for long periods throughout the year. Perhaps I will find it useful in the future. The following is a description of light therapy from *Consumers Guide to Depression:*

> The absence of full-spectrum light—light that contains all of the wavelengths of natural sunlight—can cause **Seasonal Affective Disorder (SAD)**, a form of depression which typically develops during fall and winter and goes away during late spring and summer. In about half of mild or moderate cases of SAD, symptoms can be effectively treated by *light therapy,* a treatment that exposes patients to a type of full spectrum light which compensates for daylight loss. Check with your mental health professional about the type of light source to use for this treatment. For further information use http:// www.clicshop.com.

Twenty-five

Utilize Resources of the National Alliance for the Mentally Ill

I would strongly recommend to any person who has a mental illness and their family to seek out the help of the local affiliate of the National Alliance for the Mentally Ill (NAMI). NAMI's purpose is to raise awareness about mental illness, work to advocate at that national level to increase funding for mental health services and to work towards reducing the stigma associated with mental illness. All fifty states have a regional office and normally, several affiliates throughout the state. They can advise those in need of assistance with local services such as psycho-social clubs, support groups, educational programs and housing. They serve as a clearing house for the many questions that one would have as a person with mental illness, as well as their friends or family members. I have been a volunteer with NAMI for nineteen years. It is made up of over 95 percent volunteers, mostly people with a family member who had mental illness. They reach out to help others with similar challenges.

Summary:

I'm sure there are other ways that one can discover to help their way out of depression into joy. I have suggested some ways that have helped me out of four such episodes in my life. I'm not completely over this last one following the death of my wife Ann. I feel certain I'm presently doing many of the right things to help myself, along with taking an average amount of medication (15 mg. Remeron daily). I hope I will feel ready to wean off this medication some day soon as I have in my other episodes.

I do hope some part of my suggestions will be helpful to others who are being challenged in their hope to move from depression to joyful living.

Bibliography
(Listed Alphabetically)

Andreason, Nancy, M.D., PH.D. *The Golden Age of Neuroscience*—National Alliance for Research on Schizophrenia and Depression (NARSAD)—(Volume 14—Issue 3, Fall 2002), 60 Cutter Mill Rd., Suite 404, Great Neck, N.Y., 11021. Phone 1-800-829-8289.

Bouricius, Jean K. *Psychotoxic Drugs Legal and Illegal and Psychoactive Drugs and Their Effects on Mentally Ill Persons*—National Alliance for the Mentally Ill of Western Mass., Inc. 717 ½ Main Street, Agawam, MA 01001.

Campaign For America's Mental Health—http://www.nmha.org in factr/facts sheets/21.Cfm 12/6.03.

Crack, Dinah—address unknown.

DeRoppe, Robert. *The Master Game*, Dell Publishing Co., 1968.

Discover Magazine, http://www.hasp.web.org/members only test/cgextradepression. Asp.

Falkenberg, Judy. *Using Drugs to Lift the Veil of Depression*. Food and Drug Administration Consumer, U.S. Dept. of Health and Human services, (5600 Fishers Lane, Rockville, MD 20857. Oct. 1983 Families for Depression awareness Helping Someone Who Is Depressed, http://www.familyaware.org Phone 617-924-9383.

Families for Depression Awareness (Phone 1-617-924-9388).

Fitzgerald, Scott. *The Crack Up*. New Directions Publishing Co. http://www.ndpublishing.com.

Hales, Diane, Why Prayer Can Be Good Medicine–*Parade* Magazine, 3/23/04.

Hales, Diane, Too Tough to Seek Help–*Parade* Magazine, 6/20/04.

The Healthy Heart, The Holyoke Medical Center, 575 Beech St. Holyoke, MA 01040. Phone 413-534-2789.

Jaffe, D.J.M.D. National Alliance for the Mentally Ill, 381 Park Ave. South, N.Y., N.Y., 10016. Phone 212-684-3264, or 1-800-950-NAMI. *An Overview of Electroconvulsive Therapy (ETC)*. by Dimitris Popolus, Montefiore Medical Center, posted by D.J. Jaffe, M.D. for N.A.M.I.

Mediterranean Diet, http://www.diet4uonline.com, 3/28/04.

National Institute of Mental Health—6001 Executive Blvd., Room 8184, MSC, 9663 Bethesda, MD 20892-9663.

The National Mental Health Assoc. Tel. 1-800-969-NMHA.

Rahner, Karl—Quoted from—*When God Says No,* by Father Daniel Lanahan, OSM, published by Lantern Books: http://www.lanternbooks.com. Hohokus, NJ.

The Symptoms of Depression—National Mental Health Association, 1021 Prince St, Alexandria, VA. 22314-2971. Phone 1-800-969-NMHA (1997).

Texas Christian University Daily Skiff, http://www.tcu.edu, page 25.

Utrich, Roger, Ph.D. *Redbook* Magazine, May 2004, p. 63. www.redbookmagazine.com.